INTERMITTENT FA

MW01088944

By Robert Paxton

FREE Bonus
FREE BOOK: PERSONAL TRAINER HACKS, CARDIO
Has been added to the back of this book

Introduction

Have you ever tried a low -calorie diet?

Did you get everlasting results?

Or did you find the weight eventually crept back on?

If so, **YOU NEED THIS BOOK!**

Being overweight my entire childhood, all of my teenage years, and the better part of my 20's led me to try some outrageous diet and exercise strategies. Ultimately, these equated to little to no results and almost always weight regain. I understand how disheartening it is to get yo-yo results. It's not easy to stick to eating plans. They require food prep, special foods and Navy Seal like discipline. While the professionals bicker over low carb vs balanced, keto vs vegan, and whether it's as simple as calories in – calories out, the average person is left disoriented, fed up and struggling to see any type of result. This book is going to change that!

This book includes:

- ⬚ A beginner's guide to the 16:8 method

- ⬚ Your first 30 Days

- ⬚ Why Low-Calorie Diets Make You Fat

- ⬚ The Best Exercise for Weight Loss

- ⬚ **The Third most IMPORTANT Factor Other Than Diet & Exercise Most Programs Neglect**

Thank you again for purchasing my book. Let's jump start your health & fitness goals NOW!

Contents

Chapter 1 Intermittent Fasting (IF): What is it?

What exactly does intermittent fasting refer to? Almost all of us are familiar with the word fasting. The reasons people fast vary from one group to another. For some, it is a religious practice; they sacrifice food to commit to prayer. Others have no reason; they just lack food. In past societies, people would go out to the fields to work, and eat only when they rested.

Intermittent fasting is not among the fasting practices described above. It is neither a religious practice, nor is it driven by the lack of time or food - it is a choice. It is best described as an eating pattern that alternates between eating periods and fasting periods, with each period lasting a predetermined amount of time. For example, the 16:8 method has a fasting period of 16 hours and an eating period of 8 hours.

Note that it is not a diet but an eating pattern. Less is said about the foods you should eat, but more emphasis is put on when you eat them. Does this mean you can eat whatever you want? Unfortunately not. Just like anything else in life, you're going to get out what you put in. Clean eating is one of the three factors in the tripod to fat burning success. Does this mean you must live on chicken and broccoli? No of course not. We are humans and I believe in enjoying life, but as you already know moderation is the key here.

It is important to know that IF isn't some program that popped up from somewhere, will trend for a while, and disappear like most weight loss programs do. It has been around for a long time and has been popular for many years (even if you are learning about it just now). It is one of the leading health and fitness trends in the world today. It is recommended by a range of health and fitness experts, such as the authors of "THE COMPLETE GUIDE TO FASTING" by Dr. Jason Fung and Jimmy Moore.

Let us learn more about how intermittent fasting works in the following chapter.

How is energy burnt?

Intermittent fasting has been tried and found to be a powerful fat burning and weight loss tool. But how exactly does it work? Before delving into how IF works it's important to understand some key factors:

- ☐ How the body stores energy

- ☐ How the body uses energy

- ☐ Your hormones role in this process

The body is either in a state of storing energy or burning energy. There is no middle ground.

What does this mean? Well basically if you're not burning glucose (sugar) you're storing it as either glycogen or fat. Does this mean you need to be constantly working out? Short answer- no. In fact, exercise is only 10% - 15% of the weight loss equation (more about that later). Your body burns energy in a variety of different ways. Even when you're stationary doing absolutely nothing your body expends energy as it completes functions required for living. This is what RMR or BMR refers to. However, even though your cells might be using glucose and burning energy, any excess will be stored. This would count as a state of storage.

Wait! If we're either storing sugar or burning it, logic would dictate less food and more exercise equals weight loss. It seems straight forward right? If you're reading this you have most likely tried this approach to no avail. You either saw results in the beginning only to have them come to a grinding halt or you put it all back on when you returned to your normal lifestyle.

So, how do I lose weight then?? To get a better picture we need to understand two principles:

1. How glucose (sugar) is stored and burned, or used for energy.

2. Our hormones role in this process

How is energy stored?

The body can store energy in two ways; glycogen and fat.

Food (yum) is broken down into a variety of different macronutrients through digestion. These macronutrients are absorbed into the bloodstream and transported throughout the body to our cells to use for various functions. For example, Carbohydrates are broken down into Glucose (sugar), absorbed by the blood stream and sent to cells to use for energy. However, if there is excess glucose in the bloodstream (high blood sugar), it will be stored as glycogen through a process called Glycogenesis. The body can only store so much glycogen. Once these stores are full any excess glucose is stored as fat through a process called Lipogenesis.

How is energy used?

When our cells require more energy than the bloodstream can provide (low blood sugar) glycogen is turned back into glucose through a process called glycogenolysis. Our glycogen stores are slowly emptied to raise our blood sugar levels back to normal. When these stores are empty, fat will be broken down for energy in a process called lipolysis. Now we're burning fat Wahoo!

Summary

- Excess glucose will be turned into glycogen for storage, triggered by high blood sugar
- Once glycogen stores are full, excess glucose will be turned into fat for storage
- When blood sugar levels drop, glycogen will be turned back into glucose and added to the bloodstream
- When glycogen stores are emptied, fat will be broken down and released into the bloodstream for energy

Now you have a rough idea of how and why the body stores and uses energy, we will look at some key hormones that control this process.

Hormones

Commonly associated with mood, hormones also play a huge role in your ability to lose weight. Their secretion from various glands is triggered for a variety of different reasons. For example, insulin is released by the pancreas when blood sugar levels rise. We will cover the key hormones you need to know about when it comes to weight loss.

Insulin

Trigger: Produced when blood sugar rises

Mission: Lower blood sugar

Method: Insulin helps transport glucose into cells for energy. Any excess will be taken to the liver where insulin will stimulate the liver to start making glycogen.

Note: When you eat, blood sugar will rise. This rise in blood sugar will trigger a release of insulin. This is normal and important! However, constant over eating and unnecessary grazing, especially of carbohydrates, means we will constantly be spiking our blood sugar. Constant blood sugar spikes mean constant insulin secretion and because one of insulin's main functions is promoting storage, having this bad boy in your blood stream constantly means you're in a state of storage. If we continue this route for long enough we will develop what is called **insulin resistance**. This means insulin doesn't work effectively as our body has built a level of immunity to it. Now, extra insulin must be released to try and combat high blood sugar levels. With all this extra insulin in the blood stream your body will be in a storage state overload, prompting the liver to make glycogen and fat quicker than ever!

Glucagon

Trigger: Released when blood sugar drops

Mission: Raise blood sugar

Method: Glucagon stimulates the liver to break glycogen back down into glucose for the blood stream. Glucagon also plays a part in stimulating adipose tissue (fat tissue) to break down fat stores for the blood stream.

Note: As you can see, glucagon does the opposite of insulin. Having this bad boy in your bloodstream is going to help your body switch to an energy burning state.

Human Growth Hormone (HGH)

Trigger: The release of HGH is controlled by two other hormones. To keep things simple, we will leave them nameless for now. From a weight loss perspective related to fasting, all you need to know is HGH can be triggered by adequate sleep (more on this later), exercise, and low blood sugar levels.

Mission: This depends on many factors. For example, as a child HGH helps with bone growth (height) but as an adult this is not the case. To keep it relative to weight loss HGH helps regulate low blood sugar and grow muscle among many other functions.

Method: To help regulate low blood sugar levels HGH helps stimulate adipose tissue to break down stored fat for the blood stream. If you're on a weight loss journey, you want to nurture the production of this bad boy.

Note: According to the Society of Endocrinology, when the brain senses insulin-like growth factors or excessive HGH in the body it suppresses the release of HGH. They explain the method of diagnosing over production of HGH is done by giving a person a sugary drink. This should promote HGH levels to drop. What does this mean for your weight loss? Well, high glucose levels suppress the release of HGH. This means high consumption of carbohydrates and sugary foods are not only going to give you high blood sugar, but they will suppress the release of HGH meaning this hormone won't stimulate adipose tissue to break down stored fat. It also means HGH won't be in the system to stimulate muscle growth and bone density.

Leptin

Trigger: Leptin is released by fat cells. The more fat cells you have, the more leptin released.

Mission: Leptin helps stabilize weight by regulating hunger, satiety, and appetite.

Method: Leptin levels relate to how much body fat you have. The more body fat, the more leptin in the blood stream. The less body fat you have, the less leptin your blood stream will have.

Note: When losing weight, the drop in body fat will lead to a drop in leptin levels. This results in an increase of appetite. Understanding this will help you understand why losing weight sometimes makes you feel like you want to eat a horse! Like insulin, the body can develop leptin resistance. When overweight, the extra amounts of leptin in the bloodstream can cause the body to build an immunity, meaning even though you carry a lot of body fat, the leptin doesn't work effectively to suppress your appetite. This can stimulate over eating and imbalance of the previously mentioned hormones.

Ghrelin

Trigger: Known as the hunger hormone, ghrelin levels in the blood rise just before eating time. The timing of this rise correlates to your normal eating routine.

Mission: Ghrelin is responsible for a few things but to keep it simple its mission is to promote you to eat.

Method: Acts on the hypothalamus promoting appetite

Note: Ghrelin will rise in correlation with your normal eating pattern but the interesting thing is, it comes in waves. Dr Fung found that over a prolonged period without food (fasting) ghrelin levels actually drop, and hunger pangs pass. Have you ever felt hungry at lunch but were too busy to eat? Then, by the time you came to eat you weren't actually hungry any more? If you ignore the hunger pangs they will pass. Contrary to popular belief, the hunger will not keep building to unmanageable levels. It will in fact pass. After time, Ghrelin releases get less frequent or switch to the new eating pattern. This has been found to help stop cravings for sugar also.

Summary

- Insulin is a storage hormone responsible for lowering high blood sugar

- Insulin stimulates fat storage

- Glucagon is a storage burning hormone responsible for raising low blood sugar

- Glucagon stimulates the breakdown of stored fat

- Human growth hormone or HGH helps promote lean muscle mass, bone density and the breakdown of stored fat

- HGH is a burning hormone (among other functions) responsible for raising low blood sugar

- HGH is suppressed by insulin, high blood sugar, and eating carbohydrates

- Leptin suppresses hunger

- The more body fat you have the more leptin your blood stream has

- High amounts of leptin can cause resistance meaning even though you have a high body fat percentage, you may still feel hunger and over eat

- Ghrelin promotes hunger

- Eating can spike ghrelin; making you hungry

- Ghrelin release lowers the longer you go without food

- Ignoring hunger long enough will make the need to eat pass

So How Exactly Will IF Help You Burn Fat?

Your fasted period is going to promote:

1. Lower insulin levels because there is no incoming food. This means insulin won't be stimulating the liver to store glycogen and fat

2. Lower blood sugar triggering the release of glucagon and HGH. These hormones will promote the breakdown of glycogen and fat stores, to raise blood sugar and supply energy

3. The breakdown of fats for energy will promote fat burning

4. Increased levels of HGH will help maintain muscle during the fat burning process

5. Lower body fat percentage helps to combat leptin resistance

6. Slowly suppress ghrelin secretion which will stop hunger, sugar cravings, and overeating

Your eating period is going to:

1. Supply the body with vital nutrients

2. Keep you sane because life is short and food is awesome!

Hopefully you can see that it is in fact hormone imbalance that prevents you getting the results you seek. In order to burn fat, we must first burn glycogen. Factors such as constant insulin spiking or insulin resistance heavily affect our ability to tap into stored fat. This is why you will often find little results no matter how hard you work out. If these key hormones aren't stimulated effectively you will struggle to gain everlasting results.

Why Low-Calorie Diets Don't Work

Have you ever tried lowering your calories to lose weight? Did it work long term? Could you keep the weight you lost off? If you're reading this book, my guess is that it didn't, and you're not alone. Data from the UK show 1 in 124 obese women get results using this method, meaning the nutrition guidelines some professionals are following have a 99.5% fail rate. A quick goggle of what happened to the contestants on the hit TV series "The Biggest Loser" should be enough to put you off this method. This show is a classic example of why moving more and eating less only works in the short term, if at all. There is a reason there are few reunion shows. So why are low calorie diets flawed?

A study on 14 contestants on the biggest loser show revealed some alarming results six years after filming had finished. The initial results were impressive but as the study showed, they were short lived. Below are results of some of the factors tested.

Weight

- **Average weight before filming: 328 lb/ 148 kg**

- **Average weight after 30 weeks on *the show:* 199 lb/ 90 kg**

- **Average weight six years after final: 290 lb/131 kg**

As you can see, contestants lost a massive amount of weight during filming, but struggled to maintain the weight loss over a long period of time.

One of the 14 who participated in the study managed to keep the weight off. That's over a 95% fail rate! So why is this?
Check out the results below showing contestants Resting metabolic rate (RMR).

Resting Metabolic Rate

RMR reflects the amount of energy or calories
the body burns to stay alive without movement.
In some places this is measured in BMR or basal metabolic rate.
RMR is responsible for around 70% of your entire
metabolism which is why the results below are shocking.

- **Average RMR before filming: 2,607 kcal burned / day.**
- **Average RMR after 30 weeks on the show: 1,996 kcal burned / day.**
- **Average RMR six years after final weigh-in: 1,903 kcal burned / day.**

As you can see, even though contestants put around 70% of their initial weight back on, their RMR did not raise back to its levels pre-filming. It stayed around 700 calories lower a day! This means to lose the same amount of weight second time round, contestants would need to eat 700 less calories than they did on the show. Considering the original diet consists of 1200 - 1500 calories with 90 minutes of exercise six days a week. This would be near impossible. So why did the contestants RMR stay so low even when they put the weight back on?

Metabolic adaptation

I mentioned BMR (basal metabolic rate) and RMR (resting metabolic rate) earlier. These both refer to how much energy (calories) your body uses to live without action and make up roughly 70% of your entire metabolism. When you sit in caloric deficit, the bodies BMR/RMR will slowly drop as it enters starvation mode, meaning it will burn less calories. Basically, your metabolism slows down. This is an important reaction through times of famine. The body doesn't want to use its stored energy, and naturally uses incoming energy sparingly. This is not beneficial when the aim is everlasting, sustainable weight loss. When you start dieting in this manner and increase your exercise you will generally only see results at the start before your body's metabolism adjusts for the lack of food. Once it adjusts, your results become stagnant and often times after frustration people give up and all the weight comes piling back on. If you're lucky your RMR/BMR will rise with the weight gain, ensuring you only end up putting back on what you lost, but constant yo-yo dieting could lead to a lower metabolism meaning you will struggle to lose weight and could even end up the heaviest you've ever been!

So, if eating too little causes this, you're probably wondering how not eating at all over a period of time could be any better right? Keep reading to see why.

Intermittent fasting vs Low calorie diets

Low calorie diets simply don't cause the hormone adaptations fasting does. Remember those hormones we covered earlier in the book? They are the key to weight loss and your salvation. Remember how we need the help of hormones such as glucagon and HGH to stimulate the liver and fat cells to break down stored energy? As we now know they're triggered by low blood sugar levels. This is accomplished during the fasted period. Other hormones I haven't mentioned for simplicity's sake are also stimulated during this window to prevent metabolism drops associated with low calorie diets. Low calorie diets still include eating, and every time we eat our blood sugar levels are going to rise which triggers.........Insulin! As you now know, insulin is a storage hormone. So even though you might be consuming low calories, your lowered metabolism plus this little guy equals stored fat. Nothing turns off HGH like high blood sugar levels and insulin which ruins your chance to maintain muscle mass.

Summary

- Low calorie dieting could ruin your metabolism making maintainable weight loss near impossible

- Maintainable weight loss relies heavily on hormone adaptation

- Fasting stimulates key hormones for metabolism retention, muscle preservation, and fat burning

Chapter 2 Intermittent Fasting: 16:8 Method

There are different methods of practicing IF. However, they all have a similarity; they all include a feeding period and a fasting period.

▢ *The fasting period* – it varies in time length for the various methods. During this time, you either eat nothing at all or zero calorie beverages.

▢ *The feeding period* – it also varies in time length for each method. During this time, you may eat whatever you want in moderation to avoid overfeeding. It is advisable that you eat 'normally' and not as if compensating for the period you went without food. Some methods like The Warrior Diet may require that you eat foods in a certain order.

Before we look at the 16:8 method, it is important to point out that intermittent fasting is not for everyone. Below are some people who should not try intermittent fasting:

▢ Children

▢ People with diabetes (both type 1 and 2) without first seeing a doctor

▢ Pregnant and breastfeeding mothers

▢ People with eating disorders

▢ People with low body fat

▢ People under 18

▢ People with high cortisol levels

WARNING: Before undertaking any diet, physical exercise program or change to your normal habits you should see a doctor or other relevant professional.

Keep it safe guys!

Let us now look at the 16:8 method specifically.

16 8 The Lean gains protocol

As the name suggests, this method is divided into two periods; a 16-hour fasting period and a specific 8-hour feeding period. It is important that you keep your feeding period constant. This means that you cannot decide to eat from 8am to 4pm today and shift it to 8pm to 4 am the next day. This is for the sake of creating a schedule that is easy for your body to adapt to and easy to follow. Remember the hunger hormone ghrelin is released in correlation with your eating pattern? Changing your pattern constantly could leave you hungry all the time and play havoc with the hormones we mentioned.

This method is said to be more sustainable and easier to stick to as you are not required to go to long without food, and it can easily fit into most people's day to day lives. For instance, the average person sleeps for eight hours. You only need to fast for 8 more hours while awake, which makes the fasting period seem shorter.

For example, if your last meal was at 10pm, you fast until 2pm the following day some, of which you will be asleep, and the rest busy at work - you will barely notice the time. This method is popular as you can still have dinner with family or friends before your feeding window closes.

Important Note: Some research suggests eating late at night produces higher insulin spikes than during the day impacting sleep quality and promoting storage overnight.

As you probably know, nutrition plays a big role in any health and fitness journey. The thing is we often know what to eat! You know vegetables are good for you, meat has protein, and you probably know processed food is generally bad. I'm not going to give you the same old avoid bread, pasta blah blah spiel you've heard a hundred times. However, we will cover two essential electrolytes vital to your weight loss people arc often lacking as well as how many fats, proteins and carbs you should consume for the best results.

Note: In the beginning just focus on getting used to your window. You will get immediate results. Once you are used to the 16:8 lifestyle move on to more advanced concepts for further results.

Fats, Carbs & Protein

As mentioned before, the aim of the game is to burn through glycogen stores forcing the body to use fat. Over time the aim is to get our body used to burning fat as its' primary fuel source to keep lean all year round. The best way to do this is to restrict carbs and increase fat consumption. It's worth noting that protein should be kept at a moderate level as too much can be converted into glucose and stored by the body as glycogen. Below are some examples of common macros. I want to take this opportunity to note you don't have to be Keto or following a ketogenic diet to get results with IF.

Always make sure to consult your doctor before changing your diet.

Fat: 50%
Protein: 30%
Carbohydrates: 20%

Fats: 60%
Protein: 30%
Carbohydrates: 10%

Fat: 65%
Protein: 25%
Carbohydrates: 10%

Protein Guidelines

A common mistake when trying to lose weight is eating too much protein. As mentioned earlier, excess protein can be converted to glucose (sugar) and stored as glycogen. Due to the difference in atomic makeup, glucose cannot be converted back into protein. Below are some guidelines you can follow depending on your goal.

Weight loss = 0.36g – 0.7g per pound of <u>TARGET</u> body weight.

Example: Mandy weighs 198lb but has a goal weight of 174lb.
0.36 x 174 = 62.64
0.70 x 174 = 121.8

Mandy's ideal daily intake of protein is 62g – 122g.
Mandy would now make sure she had at least 62g of protein per day to preserve muscle, but eat no more than 122g per day to avoid having protein converted to glucose.

Bulking = 1.5g – 2g per pound of <u>TARGET</u> body weight.

Example: John weighs 165lb but has a goal weight of 200lb.
1.5 x 165 = 247.5
2 x 165 = 330

John's ideal daily intake of protein is going to be 247g – 330g.
John is most definitely going to need supplements as the amount of food needed to achieve this amount of protein can be unbearable to eat. When bulking, it is common for body fat percentage to increase but once the goal weight is achieved a cutting phase would be implemented.

Carbohydrate Guidelines

Calculating carbohydrates can be tricky, as it differs from person to person. Below are some guidelines you can follow.

Keto = 30g or less per day.
These should come predominately from leafy greens. This method is a principle taken from the ketogenic diet.

Plateau buster = 100g or less per day.
These should come predominately from leafy greens and resistant starches. This principle is handy if you have hit a plateau.

Beginner = Eliminate refined sugars.
Rather than focusing on macros, the beginner's focus should be on eliminating refined sugars and incorporating resistant starches.

Resistant Starches

Are resistant to digestion and function like a soluble fiber. They help lower blood sugar levels and insulin resistance among other things. These are better choices than traditional carbohydrate choices.

Examples:

Sweet potato & yams instead of potatoes
Oats instead of cereal
Cooked & cooled rice instead of warm rice
Green bananas instead of other fruit

Fat Guidelines

Some people still find it hard to comprehend that consuming fat does not automatically transfer to "getting fat".

As Nina Teicholz reveals in her book *The Big Fat Surprise*, the low-fat movement is full of misinformation and shady scientific support. I highly suggest you check Nina and her book out.

If you want to burn fat as fuel to attain everlasting weight loss, you will have to come to terms with eating more fat than you may have thought healthy. I'm not saying you have to go keto, but a steady intake of saturated fats will help your body transition to burning fat as fuel.

AVOID Trans- Fat & Hydrogenated Oils

Partially hydrogenated oils contain trans-fat. Trans fat causes a host of different health problems including the rise of LDL ("bad") cholesterol.

Eat Saturated Fat

Fully hydrogenated fats become saturated fats. The difference? They contain no trans-fat. If it stays solid at normal room temperature its safe to assume its saturated fat.

Examples of healthy fats

Avocado
Fatty Fish
Extra Virgin Olive Oil
Coconut Oil
Full Fat Yogurt
Nuts
Whole Eggs
Cheese

Cooking Guidelines

Saturated fat is the safest substance to cook in. Unlike other fats and oils, saturated fat does not become hydrogenated under heat.

Quick Tips

AVOID cooking in vegetable and soy bean oils as they are hydrogenated oils.

Although olive oil is a healthy form of fat when cold, when heated it becomes partially hydronated. Use for dressings but NOT for cooking.

Remember, if it's solid at normal room temperature it's most likely saturated fat. Any fat that remains a liquid at normal room temperature (even the healthy ones) will become hydrogenated under heat.

Dairy & Animal Products

Provided you aren't allergic or vegan, animal products are a great way to meet your protein and fat requirements. However, there's a few things you should take into account when consuming them.

As Dr.Gundry explains in his book *The Plant Paradox,*
What our food ate can affect us! If your avoiding grains to lose weight but still chowing down on grain feed animals you could be in for a host of health problems rather than a Instagram worthy beach bod.

Dr. Gundry explains grass feed beef has a natural balanced ratio of omega-6 to omega-3 fats which is 3:1. Perfect for us he proclaims. Too much omega-6 can cause health problems which kick in around a ratio of 4:1. Gundry explains some grain feed beef can have a ratio of up to 20:1......Wow moment!

Animals like cows did not evolve to eat grains and are pumped with drugs to stop them feeling the ill effects it has on their bodies. Companies do this to save money...Inhumane and bad for your body.

Check out Dr. Gundry's book **The Plant Paradox**. It is an amazing read!

Fruit Guidelines

There's so much conflicting information about fruit that it deserves a special mention in this book.

The simple fact is **FRUIT IS HIGH IN SUGAR.**

On the molecular level your cells do not divide foods like fruit and chocolate into "healthy" and "not healthy" category's. Glucose is glucose, period. Any other form of sugar, fructose, dextrose and any other word ending in "ose" is converted to glucose and used accordingly.

Fruit should only be eaten in season and in very small amounts if you are trying to lose weight. Our bodies are wired to use fruit as a bulking agent for the colder months when food will be scarce. Our bodies don't realize that we live in a society where we have access to food all year round. By constantly eating fruit your telling your body that it should be moving into a state of storage because winter is coming.....

Here is how I recommend you use fruit when trying to lose weight

- Ditch fruit smoothies
- Consume fruit straight after workouts with a protein shake
- Never eat fruit without a source of protein

Fruit smoothies are sugar bombs. The amount of sugar cancels out any antioxidant effects the drink may have. Use leafy green smoothies instead for the same benefits. Consuming fruit after workouts with a protein shake is a great way to spike insulin so the muscle cells can absorb the protein shake. I know spiking insulin is usually a red light when fasting for weight loss but in this instance, it will promote lean muscle gain because Insulin is also responsible for helping cells absorb protein. If you're going to eat fruit as a snack make sure to eat it with a protein source such as nuts. This will slow the sugars absorption into the bloodstream, giving you longer lasting energy and preventing energy loss later in the day.

Breakfast Guidelines

Another controversial topic that deserves a special mention is breakfast. You've probably heard that breakfast is the most important meal of the day. This is totally true but.....

YOU DON'T HAVE TO EAT BREAKFAST IN THE MORNING.

The word breakfast simply means break your fast. Break – Fast.
From now on just think of breakfast as your first meal of the day regardless of what time you eat it. For example, I have breakfast at 1pm - 2pm. Traditionally people find 16:8 easier by starting their eating window later in the day. This isn't gospel....Pick whatever window suits you. So if you're a person who hates eating in the morning don't worry, that's not the reason you can't lose weight.

The biggest tip I can give you when it comes to your first meal is.....

Make sure it's high in protein and fats but low in carbohydrates.
The reason for this is whatever you eat first will determine what fuel your body will burn over the course of the day. A high carbohydrate breakfast will prime the body to seek sources of sugar giving you nasty sugar cravings, energy dips and foggy brain. A breakfast full of protein and fats will prime the body to seek fat for fuel, and keep you fuller for longer. Starting the day with this kind of breakfast has also been shown to help with anxiety and depression by promoting higher levels of serotonin.

So....

- Ditch fruit smoothies for leafy green alternatives
- Ditch cereals for foods like eggs and avocado
- Feel free to drop a bit of grass feed meat into the mix
- Avoid resistant starches in this meal also

Summary

- Use the formula listed under protein guidelines to accurately calculate your daily protein needs
- Resistant starches are better for blood sugar levels and promote insulin sensitivity
- Cooking with saturated fat is healthier than using hydrogenated oils such as vegetable oil
- It's saturated fat if it stays solid at normal room temperature
- Grain feed animal products are inhumane and unhealthy
- Fruit can promote storage
- Eating fruit without a protein source spikes blood sugar and insulin
- Breakfast simply means break your fast
- Not eating in the morning will not keep you fat
- Your first meal should be high protein and fat

Electrolytes

These bad boys contribute to many different functions in our bodies from muscle contraction, to message sending between brain and organs. To give you the best possible start without overwhelming you, I'm going to talk about two important electrolytes you can start adding to your diet TODAY.

Potassium

Muscle Cramps & Tightness

When we get muscle cramps we are commonly told we lack water and/or magnesium. Now this is true, but another reason for muscle tightness could be a lack of potassium. This is because we need far more potassium a day than magnesium.

Some signs of low potassium can include:
- Muscle tightness
- Swollen ankles
- Sugar cravings (Yes low potassium could cause sugar cravings)

Some sources of potassium
- Beet Tops

- Avocado

- Spinach

- Lima Beans

- Potato

- Brussel Sprouts

Try adding some of these into your diet more regularly to boost your potassium. Be aware of potato and lima beans as they have a high carbohydrate content. These are best kept in moderation.

Magnesium

<u>Muscle Cramps & Tightness</u>

As you probably already know, low magnesium can cause muscle cramp. It is interesting to note that a lot of magnesium is lost from food during the digestion process. Rock salt baths and magnesium creams are a great way to make sure your muscles are getting enough.

Some signs of low magnesium can include:
- Muscle soreness
- Insomnia
- Anxiety/ depression

Some sources of magnesium:
- Spinach
- Almonds
- Quinoa
- Sesame seeds

These two electrolytes are very important, but as you can see, are easily added to your diet. Of course, there's more, but getting more of these two is a great start to burning fat! I highly recommend supplementing these two, as it can be hard to get enough through food alone.

Chapter 4 Exercise

The obvious second part to the puzzle is exercise. Exercise has many wonderful benefits. It can help with depression and anxiety, while also helping you to attain your aesthetic goals. Exercise is also going to play a part in the balancing of the hormones mentioned earlier. Exercise promotes the production of HGH, but will also help drain glycogen stores quickly.

What is the best exercise when fasting?
It is popular belief that long drawn out cardio at a steady pace is the best way to burn fat. In my experience, this is not the case. Although it has its benefits, when it comes to burning fat and the IF lifestyle, I've had far more success with HITT training for both female and male clients.

High Intensity Interval Training (HITT)
If burning fat is your mission I recommend HITT training. Fast paced workouts that can be done in 30 minutes make this ideal for someone with a busy lifestyle. HITT can be done with bodyweight exercises, barbells, kettlebells and dumbbells. I usually look to use exercises that use more than one muscle group. For example, a row rather than a bicep curl. The name of the game is short bursts at near maximum effort. Below are some guidelines you can play with. They are meant as guidelines, not gospel!

- 20 second exercise – 10 second rest (Advanced)
- 10 second exercise – 20 second rest (Intermediate)
- 10 second exercise – 30 second rest (Beginner)

Rounds:
- 8+ (Advanced)
- 3-6 (Intermediate)
- 1-3 (Beginner)

Number of exercises:
- 7+ (Advanced)
- 5-6 (Intermediate)

- ☐ 3-5 (Beginner)

Example workouts

Beginner
- ☐ **Squat**
- ☐ **Running on the spot**
- ☐ **Star Jumps**

Intermediate
- ☐ **Burpees**

- ☐ **Weighted squat**

- ☐ **Press Up**

- ☐ **Medicine Ball Slam**

- ☐ **Battle Ropes**

Advanced
- ☐ **Burpee/High Jump**

- ☐ **Box Jump**

- ☐ **Kettlebell Swing**

- ☐ **Clean & Press**

- ☐ **Battle Ropes**

- ☐ **Kettlebell Row**

Fasted Exercise

As you now know, during your fasted state blood glucose levels drop and glycogen stores are depleted. Without a ready supply of these easily available sources of energy, the body must adapt and pull from the other source of energy that is available – fat.

According to John Rowley, Wellness Director for the International Sports Science Association (ISSA), exercising when hungry has one main advantage; increasing your body's ability to burn more fat. He says, "The less glucose you have in your system the more fat you will burn."

Founder and CEO of Diet Free Life, LLC, Robert Ferguson, M.S., C.N, supports Rowley's insight. He says, "Your muscles don't have much sugar to draw from so you are more likely to tap into your stored energy, which means releasing and burning what I refer to as surplus fat,"

After exercising while hungry, it is recommended that you have a post workout meal, which means that you should schedule your meal to fall an hour or so after your workout. Most of the food that you consume will not be stored as fat, as it normally would. Most of it will be burned as energy to aid in the recovery process.

Chapter 5 Recovery, Rest & The Importance of Sleep

As promised, here is the third (perhaps most important) part of the weight loss puzzle which is often neglected. Sleep! Getting proper sleep can skyrocket your results - here's how.

Our body primarily enters an anabolic (building) type phase during sleep. Our body goes to work repairing damage, replacing cells, and believe it or not, burning fat. Shawn Stevenson explains this in his book **"Sleep Smarter: 21 Essential Strategies to Sleep Your Way to A Better Body Better Health and Bigger Success"**. This book has outlined key hormones you should know about for weight loss, but there are many more. Some help initiate repair and growth and some help keep us awake and/or alert. One of the big factors dictating the creation and release of these hormones is quality sleep. Stevenson cites studies showing sleep deprivation can be linked to high levels of hormones such as cortisol and insulin (Remember what too much insulin does?). He also mentions hormones correlated with fat burning that are only secreted during sleep and darkness. Remember how HGH helps burn fat? Quality sleep is linked to the creation of this hormone. If you're not getting quality sleep at the right times, all the exercise and healthy eating may not yield the results you were hoping for. If you've ever dieted before while thrashing yourself in the gym only to see little to no results, you know how frustrating this is! Perhaps proper sleep was the missing piece you needed!

4 tips to sleep better at night

TIP 1 – Get more sun

Our body's circadian system or "body clock" plays a huge role in the production of hormones. This is heavily influenced by sunlight. Stevenson explained Light, specifically morning sunlight, signals your glands and organs it's time to wake up, queuing them to produce day time hormones (most of these helping keep you alert and awake). If our bodies get inefficient sunlight in the morning and then too much artificial light at night (such as TV, laptops and smart phones) our circadian clock gets jumbled. This can cause our glands to produce hormones that prevent us sleeping. Lack of quality sleep is going to hinder the production of hormones such as HGH and could even spike the creation of hormones such as insulin. If this happens we won't burn fat over night!

TIP2 – Avoid screens before bedtime

If you are someone who watches TV until 11pm or falls asleep to YouTube on your phone, the quickest way to improve sleep would be to stop using your devices at least an hour before bedtime. Remember how our body clock is impacted by sunlight? It's also impacted by artificial light. Our eyes are a major light sensor and the blue light produced by our favorite screens stimulate our body to produce day time hormones which are primarily for keeping us awake and active. With these bad boys circulating our body, falling asleep will be hard and our body won't produce those sweet anabolic hormones we need to repair and lose weight. Some of which Stevenson cited as only being produced in the dark. Interesting!

NOTE: My clients often argue that watching TV or some other device helps them go to sleep and without it they toss and turn. The information above is to achieve quality sleep and even though you might feel that way, I find in most cases this is simply because the client has made this a habit. I encourage you to find other activities to replace your device, rather than lying in the dark stressing about not going to sleep.

TIP 3 – Sleep in darkness

Although this might seem apparent after the first two tips, some of my clients neglect this tip when not told. We can't control lights outside, such as street lamps and annoying security lights, but these could still affect our sleep on the molecular level, interrupting repair and leaving us tired the next day. Black out your windows with heavy duty curtains to stop pesky outside lights ruining your healing process!

P.S If it wasn't obvious turn out lamps, nightlights ect as well.

TIP 4 – Quality not Quantity

One of the most beneficial points I took away from Stevenson's book was that there is a sweet time window during the night where sleep is the most beneficial. During this window, our body produces the best number of hormones needed for repair and fat loss. He explained this was roughly between 10pm and 2am leaving every hour out of this window as a bonus. He also noted this could vary depending on time of year and what time zone you are in but suggested getting to bed as soon as possible after dark falls.

Improving your sleeping habits is key to weight loss, building muscle and living a healthier life in general. This important factor is often neglected in weight loss programs perhaps being the missing piece you needed! Quality sleep is going to ensure proper adaptation of key hormones for fat burning and might even be more important than increasing your exercise in the gym. Set a consistent bed time and make sure to get to bed about 30 to 60 minutes prior.

Chapter 6 Starting IF Your First 30 Days

3 Crucial Factors To Success

#1 Goal Setting
You must have a clear vision of what you want to achieve. Vague goals like I want to get - "fit", "healthy" or "lose a couple of pounds" just won't cut it when the going gets tough. You need a clear reason for doing this or you are most likely going to quit. When coaching clients, I tell them to consider 3 factors.

What do you want to do that you cannot currently in:
- 30 Days

- 90 days

- 12 Months

What do you want to look like in:
- 30 Days

- 90 days

- 12 Months

How do you want to feel in:

- 30 Days

- 90 days

- 12 Months

After filling this out I also tell them to ask themselves why they want these things and what they think will be different if they were to achieve these goals. This will help you realize what is actually important to you. Analyze your data and set a:

- 30 Day Goal

- 90 Day Goal

- 12 Month Goal

#2 Organization

Evaluate your schedule! I often see people choose an eating window only to find they don't have time to eat during this period. Not a good start! Also evaluate where you might struggle to go without food. For example, if you're a boredom eater it's probably not wise to set your fasted window during the slowest part of your day. If eating dinner with your family is habit, then allow for that in your eating window. Be smart when choosing your feeding window. Make this process as easy as possible for yourself.

#3 Support

It is important to surround yourself with positive people who are on the same journey. It's going to get rough and at times, you will want to quit. Having others to support you is key to success and could be the difference between you quitting or keeping up the fight!

Feel free to check out our Facebook Page: @LearnIFNow

Here you can private message us any questions you may have and join our private Facebook group for support and motivation from people on the same journey as yourself.

Week 1 – In week one you are simply going to adapt to the window.

Tasks

1. Choose your preferred eight hour eating window. Remember sleep is allocated to your fasting window. Try to base your eating window within times you feel it will be hardest not to eat and show discipline.

2. Do not change the type of food you eat drastically. This week is about getting used to the eating window.

3. Do not exercise. If you are new to fasting exercise will most probably spike hunger making discipline harder. Only focus on staying within your window.

4. Practice the 16:8 method Monday – Friday and have the weekend off.

Week 2 – If you managed to stick to the tasks outlined in week 1, move on to the tasks set out below. This week we will address sleep, and continue to practice the 16:8 eating pattern.

Tasks

1. Assess last weeks eating window. Do you need to change it? Does it fit with your schedule? If yes, continue to practice this window Monday - Friday. If no, select a new eating window and repeat week 1.

2. Implement one of the four tips for better sleep outlined earlier in this book from Monday – Friday

3. Feel free to lightly exercise if you have itchy feet! However, I would still recommend no exercise if you are struggling with hunger to allow full adaptation of your eating window.

4. Again, do not change the type of food you eat drastically.

Week 3 – This week we will add exercise. You've probably been hanging out to burn some calories if you haven't already started!

Tasks

1. Access your eating window. Is it still working? Does it need to change to help you be more disciplined? If the window is fine continue with your current window Monday – Friday. If not, select a new window and return to week 1.

2. Add appropriate HITT training based on your ability level. Using the guidelines for HITT training outlined earlier in this book, create a workout to complete two – three times this week. Remember; always consult a relevant professional before under going any diet or exercise plan. Continue to practice your selected tip for sleep quality from the previous week.

   Start cutting back sugar. This task depends on the person. Most people naturally know where they need to start!

Week 4 - By week four you should have your ideal eating window in place.

Tasks

1. Continue with your chosen eating window Monday-Friday

2. Add some of the foods outlined under electrolytes for added magnesium and potassium

3. Research healthy dessert options to help keep sane! The trick here is to find keto desserts as they will be high in fat and low in carbohydrates. Remember, fat spikes less insulin and will help your body switch to using fat for energy. Don't believe the "low fat" agenda. Feel free to check out our Facebook page under week 3 for ideas.

4. Implement a second tip for better sleep outlined in this book. (My personal favorite is more sunlight).

5. Continue to eliminate sugar

6. Perform 2-4 HITT workouts

As you can see, the first 30 days of 16:8 is not drastic. I have not outlined giving up bread, potato or even sweet treats. Your first 30 days should be spent making positive changes, and attaining great results to keep you motivated to continue. The key to long term success lays in how you start. I advise against rushing forward as a beginner, even though I know how desperate you are for results. The number one reason people give up initially is from trying too much, too soon. Sometimes, we have spent 5 – 20 years being overweight or unhealthy. It is unreasonable to expect yourself to reverse life long habits and lack of discipline in the blink of an eye!

Tips to Survive IF

Some people can go for 24 hours or more without food but for others, it is a real struggle to go for as little as six hours (Thanks grehlin). If you are in the later group, it does not mean that IF is not for you. There are a few ways to help you cope.

1. **Stay Hydrated** - sometimes our bodies interpret dehydration as hunger. You may feel those hunger pangs and think, 'Oh I need to eat something'. Sometimes all you need to do is sip something. While fasting, take lots of water. You can also drink black coffee, black tea, sparkling water and other zero calorie drinks.

2. **Stay Busy** – Have you ever been hungry at work but not had the chance to eat? Often, when you finally get the chance to eat you're not actually hungry anymore. By staying busy, you can replicate this. Remember hunger comes in waves.

3. **Give It Time** – Sometimes we get too impatient, especially when it comes to losing weight. We diet or exercise for two days then we check the scale and the mirror to see 'the big change' and then we get disappointed. What happens when you get disappointed? You fall off the wagon. If you want to get anywhere with IF, you must give it time. First, allow the eating pattern time to do its wonders to your body. You only need to keep going and the change will show itself.

4. **Give Your Body Time To Adapt To Fasting** - You just stopped eating six meals a day every day. Your body may react differently now that it has to make do with fewer meals. Hunger, headaches and sometimes body weakness are among the discomforts you may experience. Don't give up! Use logic though. Keep it Safe!

End Note

I invite you to think of your goals as a journey, this book as the start, and your goal as the finish. The roads and paths in between will vary, and be full of both victories and losses. Your humble beginning and your eventual triumph mean nothing without the winding roads that link them, and vice versa. Everyone admires those who have "made it". Whether that is in regard to weight loss, or some other human want like riches or fame. We are especially motivated by those who appear to have come from nothing or succeeded against all odds, but the road that links these two paradigms is just as important as the factors themselves. The roads are scarcely revered unless the end is reached, otherwise it is simply a road leading nowhere, a lost cause – failure. Those who have nothing or are underprivileged are seldom celebrated unless they manage to follow a path with a successful ending. Your health and fitness journey is not exempt from such parameters. You have most likely started a hundred times. You have most likely trodden many paths seeking your goal, only to find fleeting success or failure. I hope this book will arm you with enough hope to start once again and lead you on the right path to your ultimate victory, perhaps inspiring those around you to take action and do the same.

We have come to the end of the book. Thank you for reading, and congratulations for reading until the end. I hope this book has provided you with adequate information about intermittent fasting for weight loss, and what you need to do to get started. The next step is to adopt intermittent fasting and enjoy the amazing benefits this eating style has to offer..

References

Author: Shawn Stevenson
Title: **"Sleep Smarter: 21 Essential Strategies to Sleep Your Way to A Better Body Better Health and Bigger Success"**

Authors: Dr. Jason Fung & Jimmy Moore
Title: *"the COMPLETE GUIDE to FASTING Heal Your Body Through*
Intermittent, Alternate-Day, and Extended Fasting"

Author: Nina Teicholz
Title*: " THE BIG FAT SURPRISE"*

Author: Dr. Steven Gundry
Title: *"The Plant Paradox"*

Chemistry@Elmhurst:Glycogenesis,Glycogenolysisand Gluconeogenesis
http://chemistry.elmhurst.edu/vchembook/604glycogenesis.html

News Medical Life Sciences: What is Lipogenesis?
https://www.news-medical.net/life-sciences/What-is-Lipogenesis.aspx

Beach Bailey: What is lipolysis?
https://beachbaby.net/what-is-lipolysis-how-does-it-happen/

You and Your Hormones: Glucagon
http://www.yourhormones.info/hormones/glucagon/

You and Your Hormones: Growth Hormone
http://www.yourhormones.info/hormones/growth-hormone/

You and Your Hormones: Leptin
http://www.yourhormones.info/hormones/leptin/

PERSONAL TRAINER HACKS: CARDIO, A GUIDE TO THE PERFECT HEART RATE

Introduction

The biggest obstacle to weight loss is knowledge. Experts argue over which is the best way to lose weight and leave the average person hopelessly wondering around the gym floor without any proper guidance or quite frankly, hope. When one finally gives up because they're sick of busting ass and getting no results, a lot of professionals are quick to blame the persons lack of discipline, personal attributes or the programme they were following. This is not good enough!
I believe a lot of good information is surrounded in too much science and personal ego.

The truth is there are many ways to lose weight. This E book will teach you one of the many tools you can use effectively use right away.

I hope you enjoy this book!

Dedicated to your success,

Robert Paxton

Chapter One: Benefits of cardio for weight loss

Increased Metabolic Rate
Adding a cardio regime specifically tailored to you can help increase overall metabolism. This means you'll burn more energy even when you're not exercising!

Stress
A big contributor to weight gain for many people is stress. But the good news is, by adding cardio to your exercise regime you can help build your stress tolerance levels. A huge portion of our clients have suffered with high stress levels, especially from work and home life. Balancing the kids and a full-time job is demanding, but with a heightened tolerance to stress you may find you're able to hugely kickstart your weight loss goals! This could help dramatically if you're a stress eater!

Sleep and Relaxation
Life is hard enough without having to face the day tired, but sometimes getting more sleep just isn't an option. You work long hours, you have children you need to get off to school and you can't just ignore your significant other - they need attention too! Sometimes it feels like there's not enough time in the day for 8-9 hours of sleep every night. A good cardio regime can help to increase your sleep quality. Even if you are only getting 6 hours of shut eye a night, cardio can help make every sleeping moment count.

Chapter 2: Set your cardio goals specifically to you!

Chances are, if you're reading this you've done cardio. I remember walking into a gym for the first time and heading straight for the treadmill. I started with walking and then worked my way up to running. If I was feeling ambitious I'd hit the bike or cross trainer as well. The problem was after my first 5kg weight drop it stopped working. Even when I increased the pace, ate less and added more time. Frustrating!!! Why was this? Simple. I had no idea what speed or frequency I should do. Although I was moving fast I didn't have my heart rate where it should be. Below is a simple formula I learnt and now use to set all my clients heart rates, so they know exactly where it needs to be to burn fat without me. The cool thing about it is it uses your personal heart rate in relation to your predicted maximal heart rate to give you that sweet fat burning zone.

Formula
220-Age=MHR
MHR-RHR=SUM
SUM x DI% =Sum
SUM + RHR = THR

Example

A 30-year-old who has a resting heart rate of 72
220-35=185
185-72=113
113 x 75%=84.75
84.75 + 156
In this book we will be searching for 60% - 75% of your predicted max heart rate. This is the range I use with a bulk of my clients looking to lose weight, especially if they are a beginner. Therefore, we will be using 60 – 75 in our equations.

Now you know how to make any cardio specific to you! This is important as everyone is different after all!

Chapter 3: Warm up/cool down/stretch

It is important to warm up, cool down and stretch when performing any exercise. Not only does it prime your body for movement to prevent injury, but it helps put the mind in a state of readiness for the workout to come. Below are examples of warm ups I use with my clients.

Stationery Bike – 5mins
Squats – 3 x 12

Rower – 700m
Lunges – 3 x 12

Treadmill walk – 10mins

I recommend using movements that complement your ability. Always make logical decisions when attempting new movement patterns. If you are a complete beginner or suffer with any medical condition or joint/body pain, seek more advice from a relevant trained professional.

Chapter 4: 30 Day Fat Furnace

Following is a programme I have created to take you from couch junkie to losing serious weight in 30 days! This easy to follow programme will gradually allow your body to build up endurance and fitness while losing weight.

Important note: Please seek clearance from a relevant medical professional before undertaking ANY Health & Fitness regime weather that be physical, dietary or otherwise. This is especially important if you suffer from ANY medical condition or injury physical, mental or otherwise.

Week 1

	Mon	Tues	Wed	Thurs	Fri	Sat	Sun
Heart rate	Rest	65%	Rest	65%	Rest	Rest	Rest
Duration	N/A	30 mins	N/A	30 mins	N/A	N/A	N/A
Type		Bike		Bike			

Week 2

	Mon	Tues	Wed	Thurs	Fri	Sat	Sun
Heart rate	65%	Rest	65%	Rest	65%	Rest	Rest
Duration	30 Mins	N/A	30 Mins	N/A	30 mins	N/A	N/A
Type	Bike		Cross trainer		Bike		

Week 3

	Mon	Tues	Wed	Thurs	Fri	Sat	Sun
Heart rate	65%	Rest	75%	Rest	65%	Rest	Rest
Duration	40 Mins	N/A	30 Mins	N/A	40 mins	N/A	N/A
Type	Cross trainer		Bike		Cross trainer		

Week 4

	Mon	Tues	Wed	Thurs	Fri	Sat	Sun
Heart rate	75%	65%	Rest	75%	65%	Rest	Rest
Duration	30 Mins	40 mins	N/A	30 mins	40 mins	N/A	N/A
	Bike	Cross trainer		Bike	Cross trainer		

Remember to use the Karvonen method to calculate your HR percentages at the start of every week as they may change. As you get fitter your resting heart rate may drop, meaning your target heart rate will change.

End Note

Boom! It's that easy my friend.

I've outlined a simple way I find works with the least amount of science jargon possible. This method can be used for setting any working heart rate all you need is the percentage at which you want to work at.

We have both struggled at some point to find the guidance we want to lose weight, to win back our confidence and have a kick ass life. It's frustrating and sometimes painful but there's light at the end of the tunnel. If I can go from fat boy to personal trainer the skies the limit for you my friend!

Good Luck!

Dedicated to your success,

Robert Paxton

99242692R00038

Made in the USA
Lexington, KY
14 September 2018